Breakthroughs in Parkinson's Therapy

Neurodegenerative Insights and Treatment Strategies

By

Karen Brach

Table of Contents

INTRODUCTION

An important turning point in medical history is the fight against Parkinson's disease, a neurological illness that is progressive and persistent. This is a momentous time for Parkinson's disease treatment and perception, marked by unparalleled advances in medical science, technology, and our understanding of the human brain. For many years, treating this illness was mostly a reactive strategy that concentrated on symptom relief at the expense of underlying causes. But new discoveries in the field of neurodegenerative research are bringing about a new era in which it may be possible to not only manage but even dramatically change the course of the disease.

Since its first description by James Parkinson in 1817, Parkinson's disease has posed a serious threat to neurology. The tremors, stiffness, and slowness of movement that are its defining symptoms only hint at the disorder's complexity. As we now know, Parkinson's disease is a complex illness with a wide range of motor and non-motor symptoms. It is not a single, monolithic disease. Traditionally, deep brain stimulation (DBS) and medications like levodopa have been the mainstays in the fight against Parkinson's disease. Although these treatments are helpful in managing symptoms, they are not curative and may eventually lose their effectiveness or cause serious negative effects.

The increasing acknowledgement of these constraints and the expanding potential of scientific investigation gave rise to the demand for a paradigm change. New developments in molecular biology, neuroimaging, and genetics are not only shedding light on possible therapy avenues but also offering deeper insights into the disease's causes. This change affects millions of people worldwide who have been diagnosed with Parkinson's disease, their families, and caregivers. It is not just a scientific breakthrough; it is deeply personal.

The paradigm change is complex, involving developments in a number of fields:

From Symptom Management to Disease Modification: Therapies that aim to slow the progression of the disease are becoming the focus of research and treatment. These include stem cell therapies, which have the ability to repair damaged neurons, and gene therapies, which try to correct underlying genetic defects.

Precision medicine: More individualized treatment regimens are possible when the genetic and environmental causes of Parkinson's disease are recognized for each patient. By adjusting interventions to the patient's unique condition, this method improves results and lowers negative effects.

Technology and Rehabilitation: The use of technology in treatment plans, ranging from virtual reality platforms that provide stimulating rehabilitation exercises to wearable devices that track symptoms and modify medicine dosages in real time, promises to improve the quality of life for Parkinson's patients.

Holistic and Integrative Care: Treatments that address a patient's physical, emotional, and cognitive needs are becoming more and more popular. This includes alternative therapies like acupuncture and mindfulness meditation, as well as nutritional therapy and psychological support.

Encouraging Patients and Caregivers: The new

paradigm acknowledges that patients and their caregivers play a crucial part in helping to manage the illness. People are given the power to actively participate in their care by creating a supportive community, offering resources for improved self-management and decision-making, and facilitating communication.

The optimism of a Cure: The rekindled optimism and passionate search for a cure may be the most important part of the paradigm change. With every new finding, scientists get closer to solving the puzzle of Parkinson's disease and developing treatments that may one day make the illness extinct.

We will delve further into these revolutionary developments in "Breakthroughs in Parkinson's Therapy: Neurodegenerative Insights and Treatment Strategies." This book attempts to provide a thorough review of the current Parkinson's therapy and a glimpse into the future of treatment through interviews with top researchers, analysis of the most recent clinical studies, and firsthand accounts from those fighting this battle.

Recognizing the teamwork that is causing this change is crucial as we set out on this path. Advocates, patients, doctors, and scientists all contribute to this changing environment. Their tenacity, inventiveness, and unshakable dedication are propelling advancement in directions previously unthinkable.

There are obstacles in the way of the future. The process of converting scientific findings into practical therapies is difficult and time-consuming, and scientific advancements frequently generate more questions than they do answers. The developments covered in the upcoming chapters, however, mark a fundamental shift in our understanding of Parkinson's disease—from managing decline to promoting hope and healing. They are not only small steps forward.

Anyone affected by Parkinson's disease, whether as a patient, caregiver, medical practitioner, or just someone curious about the most recent advancements in the treatment of neurodegenerative diseases, should read this book. We are standing on the cusp of a new era where scientific advancement and human compassion will confront the gloom of Parkinson's disease. Welcome to the new paradigm for Parkinson's disease.

This introduction highlights the revolutionary shifts in treatment and attitude while outlining the history of Parkinson's therapy and its transforming journey into the present. It establishes the framework for the book's in-depth examination of these subjects.

CHAPTER ONE

Understanding Parkinson's Disease

Comprehending Parkinson's disease (PD) necessitates exploring the disease's intricate molecular and neurological foundations, identifying its diverse manifestations and phases of development, and staying up to date with the most recent findings about its causes and risk factors. With the goal of giving readers a thorough understanding of these important factors, this chapter hopes to shed light on the illness that affects millions of people worldwide.

The Neurology and Biology of Parkinson's Disease
The pathogenesis of Parkinson's disease, a

progressive neurodegenerative ailment that largely affects the motor system, is defined by the death of dopamine-producing neurons in the midbrain region known as the substantia nigra. One neurotransmitter that is essential for the efficient, well-coordinated operation of bodily motions is dopamine. Parkinson's disease is characterized by tremors, stiffness, bradykinesia (slow movement), and postural instability, all of which are brought on by dopamine depletion.

Lewy bodies, aberrant protein aggregates that form inside nerve cells that degrade function and ultimately cause nerve cell death, are linked to the loss of dopaminergic neurons in Parkinson's disease (PD). One of the main constituents of these

Lewy bodies is the protein α-synuclein, whose misfolding and aggregation are believed to be crucial to the pathophysiology of Parkinson's disease.

Signs, Phases, and the Course of the Illness

Parkinson's disease presents a complex clinical picture that differs greatly from patient to patient and can cause both motor and non-motor symptoms.

Motor Signs and Symptoms

Tremor: generally the most obvious symptom, generally originating in one of the limbs, the hand or fingers.

Bradykinesia: Slow motion that makes even easy

chores challenging and time-consuming.

Rigidity: Any area of the body experiencing tense muscles.

Impaired balance and coordination resulting in falls is known as postural instability.

Symptoms that are not motor:

Cognitive Impairment: Memory and executive function problems.

Mood Disorders: Anxiety and depression are prevalent.

REM sleep behavior disorder and insomnia are examples of sleep disturbances.

Blood pressure, perspiration, and bladder control abnormalities are signs of autonomic dysfunction.

The Hoehn and Yahr scale is commonly used to classify the five stages of Parkinson's disease progression. Stage 1 has modest symptoms limited to one side of the body, while stage 5 may result in bedridden or wheelchair-bound patients.

The Most Recent Studies on Risk Factors and Causes

Although the precise etiology of Parkinson's disease is still unknown, a mix of lifestyle, environmental, and genetic variables are thought to play a role.

Genetic Elements:

Numerous genetic mutations linked to Parkinson's disease (PD) have been found through research, including those in the LRRK2, PARK7, PINK1, PRKN, and SNCA genes. However, these genetic connections only explain a small fraction of instances, indicating that most people do not get the condition due to genetics alone.

Environmental Elements:

There is a connection between an elevated risk of Parkinson's disease and exposure to specific pollutants and environmental variables. These include living in a rural area, heavy metal exposure, and possibly pesticide exposure. On the other hand, although their possible functions in PD prevention are not fully understood, the "protective" effects of tobacco and caffeine have garnered attention. However, considering the various health hazards associated with these substances, their usage is not recommended.

Gender and Age:

The most important risk factor for Parkinson's disease is age, as the majority of cases occur beyond the age of 60. Additionally, men are almost 1.5 times more likely than women to get Parkinson's disease, though it's unclear why.

Recent studies center on the gut-brain axis's connection to Parkinson's disease, examining the ways that gut bacteria and the buildup of α-synuclein in the gut may affect brain function and even exacerbate the illness's pathology. Furthermore, research on neuroinflammation is shedding light on how the immune system's reaction to certain stimuli may hasten the degeneration of dopaminergic neurons.

Chapter TWO

Advances in Diagnostic Technology and Early Detection

A fast and correct diagnosis is the first step toward managing Parkinson's disease (PD) effectively. Significant improvements in diagnostic techniques and technology over the past few years have improved our capacity to identify Parkinson's disease (PD) earlier and more accurately. The necessity of an accurate and timely diagnosis for the best possible treatment outcomes is emphasized in this chapter, which also examines the new developments in diagnostics and the developing roles of biomarkers and neuroimaging in early detection.

Developments in Diagnostic Tools and Techniques

Parkinson's disease diagnosis has historically mainly depended on clinical observation, which involves determining whether the three main motor signs of the condition—bradykinesia, resting tremor, and muscle rigidity—are present. But these symptoms frequently appear after a substantial loss of dopaminergic neurons has already taken place, highlighting the need for more accurate diagnostic methods.

DaTscan Imagery:

The development of DaTscan (Ioflupane I 123

injection), a unique imaging technique that enables physicians to see the distribution and density of dopamine transporters in the brain, has been one of the most significant breakthroughs in the diagnosis of Parkinson's disease. This method has been useful in distinguishing Parkinson's disease from other disorders that show similarly, like drug-induced parkinsonism or essential tremor.

Screening for REM Sleep Behavior Disorder (RBD) with Olfactory Testing:

Recent studies show that REM sleep behavior disturbance and olfactory dysfunction are early non-motor indicators of Parkinson's disease (PD), occurring years before motor symptoms manifest. In order to identify those who are more likely to acquire Parkinson's disease, screening for these diseases has become an important technique for making earlier and more precise diagnoses.

The Function of Neuroimaging and Biomarkers in Early Detection

An important focus of Parkinson's research is the hunt for biomarkers, which are objective, quantifiable indicators of a biological or pathological process. Finding trustworthy biomarkers for Parkinson's disease (PD) could transform early diagnosis and disease monitoring.

Biomarkers:

Researchers are looking into a number of possible biomarkers for Parkinson's disease, such as genetic markers associated with the condition, neurofilament light chain (NfL), a marker of neuronal damage, and alpha-synuclein, a protein whose aggregates form Lewy bodies in PD brains. While there is yet no conclusive biomarker for Parkinson's disease, the quest is encouraging as a number of candidates appear capable of reflecting the start and course of the illness.

Neuroimaging

More and more advanced neuroimaging methods are being used to identify Parkinson's early symptoms, such as PET (positron emission tomography) and MRI (magnetic resonance imaging). These instruments can identify small alterations in the structure and function of the brain that occur before motor symptoms manifest. For instance, certain MRI sequences can detect changes in the substantia nigra, the area of the brain most affected by Parkinson's disease, while PET scans can evaluate abnormalities in the dopamine system.

Early and Accurate Diagnosis Is Essential for Effective Treatment

For a number of reasons, a timely and precise diagnosis of Parkinson's disease is essential. First of all, it makes it possible to start appropriate treatments to properly control symptoms, which may halt the advancement of the disease. Second, a precise diagnosis ensures that patients receive the appropriate therapeutic interventions and prevents the mishandling of other disorders that mimic Parkinson's disease.

Customizing Intervention Plans:

A more individualized approach to treatment is made possible by early discovery, taking into account the patient's individual symptoms, disease stage, and general state of health. It provides hope for changing the course of the disease by opening the door to neuroprotective medicines that may maintain dopaminergic neurons.

Improving Life Quality:

Furthermore, early diagnosis gives patients and their families the ability to plan ahead and take proactive measures to address any prospective problems. In addition, it makes educational materials and support services accessible, which contributes to preserving a better standard of living over time.

Progressing Research:

From the standpoint of research, precise and timely diagnosis improves the caliber of clinical trials for novel therapies. Researchers can speed up the discovery of viable medicines by obtaining more trustworthy data on the safety and efficiency of experimental therapies by verifying that individuals actually have Parkinson's disease (PD).

CHAPTER THREE

Conventional and Novel

Therapeutic Approaches

Parkinson's disease (PD) treatment options are as

varied as the illness itself. For many years, conventional therapies have served as the cornerstone of symptom management; however, recently developed therapies present fresh opportunities and optimism. This chapter explores both areas; it begins with a review of traditional therapy, moves on to the cutting edge of novel ones, and ends with a comparison of their efficacy and possible drawbacks.

An Overview of Conventional Parkinson's Disease Therapies

Drugs:

The main goal of pharmaceutical treatment for Parkinson's disease (PD) is to mimic or replenish dopamine, which is a neurotransmitter that is deficient in many PD patients. The preferred method for reducing side effects is still levodopa plus carbidopa. In the brain, this medicine is converted into dopamine, which momentarily restores the low levels. Important roles are also played by dopamine agonists, which imitate the actions of dopamine, and MAO-B inhibitors, which delay the breakdown of dopamine. Nevertheless, these drugs frequently become less effective with time and might have adverse effects like hallucinations and dyskinesias, which are uncontrollable movements.

Physical Medicine:

A key component of managing Parkinson's disease (PD) is physical therapy, which aims to enhance movement, balance, and general quality of life. Exercise regimens that are specifically designed to improve muscle strength, preserve flexibility, and lessen motor complaints. Methods such as LSVT BIG® training concentrate on the amplitude of movement, which is frequently diminished in Parkinson's disease.

Surgical Solutions:

Surgical procedures such as Deep Brain Stimulation (DBS) have the potential to significantly improve the lives of individuals with severe Parkinson's disease (PD) or those who are adversely affected by drugs. With DBS, symptoms including bradykinesia, stiffness, and tremor are greatly reduced by modifying neural activity in particular brain regions by the implantation of electrodes. DBS is safe, but like any surgical surgery, it has hazards. These include hardware issues and infection.

Investigating Novel Therapies

Innovative methods that target the disease's core mechanisms rather than merely its symptoms are defining the boundary of PD treatment.

Gene Therapy:

Targeting the genetic causes of Parkinson's disease (PD) using gene therapy is a novel strategy. Scientists hope to prevent future brain deterioration or restore normal function by directly introducing copies of advantageous genes into the brain. For instance, studies are being conducted to introduce genes that may be able to stop the progression of Parkinson's disease (PD) or to stimulate the production of dopamine. Although encouraging, gene therapy for Parkinson's disease is still in its early stages, and research is currently being done on its long-term safety and efficacy.

Stem Cell Utilization:

In Parkinson's disease, stem cell therapy offers hope for regenerating destroyed dopaminergic neurons. The possibility of regenerating damaged brain regions through stem cell transplantation is being investigated by researchers. Early research has demonstrated promise, with some patients reporting improvements in their motor symptoms.

There are still difficulties, though, including as the potential for unchecked cell development and the dangers of immunological rejection.

Novel Pharmacological Methods:

By focusing on symptoms that are not well controlled by existing medicines, novel pharmacological therapies seek to treat the non-dopaminergic elements of Parkinson's disease. These include drugs that treat mental disorders, enhance cognitive function, and ease sleep issues. The creation of neuroprotective medications, which avert or delay the worsening of Parkinson's disease by shielding neurons from harm, is another exciting field.

Comparative Evaluation of the Benefits and Possible Drawbacks

Efficiency:

Levodopa is one of the most successful traditional medications for controlling Parkinson's disease (PD) symptoms, especially in the early stages of the condition. But over time, their side effects become more serious and their effectiveness may decline. Though they do not stop the illness's progression, surgical alternatives like DBS provide significant symptom alleviation for people with severe Parkinson's disease (PD) or for those who are sensitive to the side effects of medication.

Although they are still in the early stages of research, emerging therapies provide the promise of more effective treatments or possibly a cure. In particular, gene and stem cell therapies may be able to target the underlying causes of Parkinson's disease (PD). Their ability to treat a wide range of symptoms and long-term efficacy, however, are still up for debate.

Adverse Reactions:

Conventional drugs frequently have a wide range of adverse effects, from minor ones like nausea and vertigo to serious ones like dyskinesias and hallucinations. Even while surgical therapies are beneficial, they come with the usual dangers associated with surgery, such as the requirement for device care and infection.

New treatments aim to reduce adverse effects by more specifically addressing Parkinson's disease. But they also come with risks of their own, like the possibility of immunological rejection in stem cell therapy or the unknowable long-term consequences of genetically modifying the brain in gene therapy.

CHAPTER FOUR
Holistic Care and Lifestyle Interventions

Lifestyle modifications and holistic care approaches have become vital supplements to conventional medical treatments in the complex management of Parkinson's disease (PD). These methods provide patients a sense of control over an illness that can frequently feel unpredictable and overwhelming by empowering them to actively participate in their care. This chapter examines how lifestyle factors such as nutrition, exercise, and diet affect the course of Parkinson's disease and how to control its symptoms. It also looks at complementary and alternative therapies and stresses the significance of tailoring lifestyle interventions to fit the needs and preferences of each individual.

The Effects of Lifestyle, Nutrition, and Exercise on the Advancement of Parkinson's Disease and Symptom Management

Nutrition:

A key component of managing Parkinson's disease is nutrition. Although there is no known diet that can prevent or cure Parkinson's disease, there are nutritional approaches that can help manage symptoms and enhance general health. A diet high in fruits, vegetables, whole grains, and lean proteins that is well-balanced can improve general health and energy levels. Flaxseeds and fish, which are high in omega-3 fatty acids, have been shown to have neuroprotective properties. Constipation, a typical problem in Parkinson's disease (PD), can also be managed with a sufficient fiber diet and adequate hydration.

According to recent study, PD sufferers may benefit specifically from some dietary components. Antioxidants, such as those in berries and leafy green vegetables, may counteract oxidative stress, which is a factor in the advancement of Parkinson's disease. In example, the Mediterranean diet may have preventive effects and has been linked to a decreased risk of neurological illnesses.

Practice:

Exercise is essential for managing Parkinson's disease (PD) and has advantages beyond physical well-being. Frequent exercise can enhance muscle strength, mobility, and balance while lowering the risk of falls and enhancing quality of life. Additionally, it has been demonstrated that exercise has neuroprotective benefits, which may halt the progression of disease.

Exercises that are aerobic in nature promote cardiovascular health; those that are strength trained add muscle; those that are stretching and flexible improve range of motion; and those that are balance-based lower the chance of falling. Programs designed specifically for Parkinson's disease patients, such as Tai Chi, yoga, and dancing courses, can also manage symptoms and offer social support.

Way of life:

A major part of controlling Parkinson's disease (PD) is making lifestyle changes, such as improving sleep hygiene and stress management. Because long-term stress can aggravate symptoms, stress-reduction methods like mindfulness, deep breathing exercises, and meditation are crucial parts of an all-encompassing care plan. REM sleep behavior disorder and other sleep disorders must be managed in order to preserve cognitive function and general health.

Alternative and Holistic Medicines

Many people with Parkinson's disease (PD) seek holistic and alternative therapies in addition to traditional medical treatments and lifestyle changes to better manage their symptoms and enhance their quality of life.

acupuncture

A crucial part of traditional Chinese treatment is acupuncture, which entails the insertion of tiny needles into certain bodily locations. Pain, sleep difficulties, mood issues, and other symptoms of Parkinson's disease (PD) have all been investigated as potential treatments. Despite conflicting scientific data, some research indicates that acupuncture may assist reduce pain and promote relaxation in order to potentially alleviate some PD symptoms.

Mindfulness & Meditation:

The potential benefits of mindfulness and meditation for PD patients' mental health have drawn attention. These techniques can aid in lowering PD-related tension, anxiety, and depression. It has been demonstrated that mindfulness meditation, in particular, enhances emotional control and quality of life in people with Parkinson's disease.

Alternative Therapies:

Additional holistic methods, including massage therapy, can improve wellbeing and relieve symptoms. Massage therapy can serve as an additional aid in the management of Parkinson's disease symptoms by easing muscle tension and promoting relaxation.

Customizing Lifestyle Changes

Since Parkinson's disease (PD) affects people differently, it is imperative to customize lifestyle therapies. To optimize the outcomes of these interventions, tactics should be customized based on the patient's unique symptoms, disease stage, and general health status.

Evaluation and Scheduling:

The best courses of action for each patient can be determined by a healthcare team consisting of neurologists, physical therapists, and dietitians after a thorough assessment. Enhancing adherence and success can be achieved by establishing concrete objectives and organizing gradual lifestyle modifications.

Including Preferences and Interests:
It is more likely that patients will stick with lifestyle treatments if they are included in activities and food choices that they love. For instance, picking workouts that you enjoy and can actually do, like walking, cycling, or swimming, can really help you keep an active lifestyle.

Observing and Modifying:
To meet the changing demands of patients with

Parkinson's disease, regular monitoring and changes are required. Holistic therapy and lifestyle interventions may need to be adjusted when symptoms worsen or change in order to continue being beneficial and maintaining the patient's quality of life.

In summary, complementary and alternative medicine can be used in conjunction with lifestyle modifications and patient-centered care to effectively manage Parkinson's disease. Patients may improve their quality of life and possibly influence the course and treatment of Parkinson's disease (PD) by concentrating on nutrition, exercise, lifestyle changes, and investigating complementary therapies. To optimize the advantages of these interventions and raise the quality of life for Parkinson's disease patients, they must be tailored to each patient's needs and preferences.

CHAPTER FIVE

The Use of Technology in Parkinson's Disease Management

The rapid advancement of technology is bringing about a fundamental revolution in the management of Parkinson's disease (PD). Technology is changing how Parkinson's is cared for and treated, from wearables that provide real-time symptom monitoring to artificial intelligence (AI) models that forecast disease progression. This chapter explores the cutting edge of technology, including virtual reality, wearables, artificial intelligence, and machine learning, and how they can improve the quality of life for people with Parkinson's disease.

Wearable Technology: Parkinson's Disease Monitoring and Management

With wearable technology offering continuous, real-time data on a patient's motor functions and symptoms, Parkinson's disease care has seen a radical shift. These devices can monitor a wide range of variables, including tremor intensity, gait patterns, and sleep quality. They can range from smartwatches to specialist sensors. A more sophisticated knowledge of the course of the disease and the efficacy of treatment is made possible by the data collection, which provides priceless insights for patients as well as healthcare professionals.

Tracking Symptoms in Real Time:

Wearable technology gives patients the ability to track their symptoms in real time, giving them more control over their health. This ongoing observation may reveal changes in symptoms to patients and caregivers, maybe pointing to the need for alterations in treatment. Furthermore, by using objective data instead of subjective symptom diaries, these devices can provide more precise and individualized care.

Management of Medication:

In addition, wearable technology is essential for managing medications. Wearables can help improve dosing regimens, improving the effectiveness of pharmacological therapies while limiting unwanted effects by linking changes in symptoms with the scheduling of medicine. With an illness where timing of treatment can have a major influence on quality of life, this exact customization of regimens is essential.

AI and Machine Learning's Role

The diagnosis and treatment of Parkinson's disease are being revolutionized by artificial intelligence and machine learning. AI systems have the ability to analyze large datasets, find trends, and forecast the course of diseases in ways that were previously impractical.

Forecasting the Course of a Disease:

Artificial intelligence (AI) models are being created to forecast the progression of Parkinson's disease, accounting for early symptoms, lifestyle, and genetic data. By identifying those who are most likely to have rapid illness development, these prediction models can potentially change the course of the disease and enable early intervention.

Customizing Therapy Programs:

Treatment strategies can be made more individualized with the use of machine learning algorithms. Through the analysis of data from wearables, medical records, and even genetic data, artificial intelligence (AI) can assist in customizing medicines to each patient's unique requirements, hence improving treatment results.

Improving the Process of Drug Development

AI is expediting the quest for novel treatments for Parkinson's disease in the field of medication development. Artificial intelligence (AI) can predict the effectiveness of proposed pharmaceuticals by mimicking the effects of chemicals on neural circuits. This can expedite the drug discovery process and accelerate the time it takes for new treatments to enter clinical trials.

Virtual Reality: An Emerging Technology for Therapy and Rehabilitation

With Parkinson's disease, virtual reality (VR) technology is creating new opportunities for therapy and rehabilitation. Virtual reality (VR)

provides patients with individualized, entertaining workouts that enhance motor function, balance, and cognitive abilities.

Improving Motor Abilities and Stability:

Virtual reality-based rehabilitation programs can replicate real-world situations that test and enhance balance and motor abilities. Virtual walking paths, for instance, can aid with gait improvement and fall risk reduction, which is a significant issue in Parkinson's patients. Because virtual reality is interactive, it promotes active engagement, which is essential for preserving freedom and mobility.

Rehabilitating Cognitive Function:

Virtual reality has use in cognitive training in addition to physical therapy. Patients can improve their attention, memory, and executive functioning through entertaining games and puzzles, addressing the cognitive components of Parkinson's that are sometimes obscured by muscular symptoms.

Social interaction and emotional well-being:
Virtual reality (VR) can also promote emotional well -being by providing a means of escape, relaxation, and social connection through multiplayer experiences. People who suffer from depression or social isolation due to Parkinson's disease may find this especially helpful.

CHAPTER SIX

Parkinson's Therapy's Future

The future of Parkinson's disease (PD) research and treatment is quite promising as we approach a new chapter in the disease's history. Innovative research avenues are revealing new information about the fundamental causes of Parkinson's disease (PD), opening the door to ground-breaking discoveries. There is promise for more effective interventions catered to the specific needs of each patient thanks to the possibilities of customized medicine and targeted therapy. It is almost impossible to exaggerate how crucial patient involvement in clinical trials and research is to improving our knowledge of and ability to treat this complicated neurological condition.

Innovative Research Pathways and the Prospect for Groundbreaking Findings The field of Parkinson's research is changing quickly thanks to interdisciplinary cooperation and creative thinking. It appears that several important research directions may open up new therapy options:

Immune modulation and neuroinflammation:

Recent research indicates that neuroinflammation

is a major factor in the pathophysiology of

Parkinson's disease. In order to potentially reduce

or stop the disease's progression, researchers are

looking into ways to modify the immune system's

reaction in the brain. Targeting particular immune

cells or pathways with immunotherapies presents

interesting opportunities for neuroprotection and

disease modulation.

Treating Alpha-Synuclein:

Since alpha-synuclein aggregation is a defining

feature of Parkinson's disease, pharmacological

intervention aimed at addressing it is very desirable. Reducing alpha-synuclein levels or stopping its misfolding and buildup are potential ways to delay the progression of the disease. Among the strategies being investigated in preclinical and clinical trials include gene treatments, small molecule inhibitors, and immunotherapies.

Regenerative Neurology and Stem Cell Treatment:
The promise for replacing lost dopaminergic neurons and restoring function in brain regions damaged by Parkinson's disease is presented by stem cell-based therapy. Even though there are still issues with cell survival and integration, continued research attempts to improve stem cell transplantation methods and maximize results.

Further research is being done on methods to promote endogenous neuroregeneration processes, which provide supplementary ways to restore neuronal function.

The Potential Benefits of Targeted Therapies and Personalized Medicine
A highly promising avenue for Parkinson's therapy is the move toward personalized medicine, which aims to customize treatments based on the distinct features and disease profiles of each patient:

Precision Medicine and Genetic Profiling:
The discovery of genetic risk factors and disease modifiers in Parkinson's disease has been made easier by advancements in genomic technologies.

By using genetic profiling, medical professionals can group patients according to their genetic heritage, allowing for more specialized interventions and individualized treatment regimens. By using this information, precision medicine techniques can match patients with treatments that are most likely to work for their unique genetic composition.

Monitoring and Predicting Treatment Response Using Biomarkers:

In Parkinson's disease, biomarkers are essential for tracking the course of the disease and the effectiveness of treatment. Clinicians can more precisely follow disease trajectories and modify therapy by discovering biomarkers linked to certain illness stages or treatment results. Biomarker-driven strategies have the potential to improve patient outcomes by enabling early intervention and proactive disease management.

Remote monitoring and digital health:

Personalized care delivery is made possible by the integration of digital health technologies, which allows for the remote monitoring of Parkinson's symptoms and treatment adherence. Treatment regimens can be modified in real time thanks to wearable technology, smartphone apps, and telemedicine platforms, which can offer insightful information about patients' everyday experiences. These technological resources improve communication between patients and healthcare professionals and enable patients to take an active role in their care.

The Value of Patients' Involvement in Research and Clinical Trials In order to spur innovation and advance the field of Parkinson's therapy, patient participation in clinical trials and research is crucial. Patients who voluntarily participate in research projects provide priceless information and perspectives that influence the creation of novel therapies and interventions.

Increasing the Rate of Therapeutic Development: The main method used to assess new treatments for Parkinson's disease for safety and effectiveness is clinical trials. In order to expedite the development and approval of potential medicines, bring them to market sooner, and benefit the larger Parkinson's community, patient participation in these trials is essential.

Improving Knowledge of Disease Mechanisms
In addition to improving therapeutic outcomes, patient participation in research projects advances our knowledge of the causes and course of Parkinson's disease. Through their involvement in genetic analysis, observational studies, and biomarker investigations, patients contribute to the understanding of the disease and the discovery of novel therapeutic targets.

Patient and Caregiver Empowerment:

Participating in research gives patients and caregivers access to state-of-the-art care, resources, and support systems. In addition to providing optimism for new treatment choices, clinical trial participation helps people with Parkinson's feel more connected to one another. Participating in research also encourages patient advocacy and raises awareness of the value of funding and support for Parkinson's disease research.

In summary, new avenues for research, tailored medicine strategies, and patient participation in studies and clinical trials all point to a bright future for Parkinson's therapy. Research, clinicians, researchers, and patients will all need to work together as we try to understand the intricacies of Parkinson's disease and create novel treatments. By working together, we can change the way Parkinson's disease is treated and improve the quality of life and outcomes for those who have this difficult neurological disease.

CONCLUSION

A fresh era of healing and hope

We are clearly at the beginning of a new era, one marked by optimism, healing, and the possibility of revolutionary discoveries, when we consider the journey through the complexity of Parkinson's disease (PD) and the advancements made in its management. In this last chapter, we review the major discoveries and developments in the field of Parkinson's therapy, examine how the field is changing, and issue a challenge for more activism, research, and innovation in the battle against Parkinson's disease.

An overview of the major discoveries and advancements in Parkinson's therapy

We have explored the many facets of Parkinson's disease in this book, from its neurological and molecular foundations to the wide range of treatment options accessible. We've looked at conventional treatments like drugs, physical therapy, and surgery, realizing how important they are for PD patients to manage their symptoms and live better lives. Additionally, we've looked into cutting-edge treatments that could change the course of the illness and open up new treatment options, such as gene therapy, stem cell therapy, and tailored pharmaceutical approaches.

Wearable technology, virtual reality, and artificial intelligence have all transformed Parkinson's care by offering previously unheard-of insights into the course of the disease, individualized treatment plans, and creative approaches to rehabilitation. By improving communication between patients and healthcare professionals and giving them a stronger sense of control over their condition, these technology tools enable patients to take an active role in their care.

Parkinson's Disease Treatment's Changing Environment and Its Effects on Patients and Caregivers

Parkinson's disease treatment is changing, and this has important ramifications for both patients and caretakers. The potential for better symptom management, higher quality of life, and eventually the possibility of disease modification grows with every new discovery. By customizing therapies to each patient's needs and genetic profile, personalized medicine techniques have the potential to completely transform the way that healthcare is delivered by increasing efficacy and reducing negative effects.

In addition, the incorporation of technology in the treatment of Parkinson's disease not only improves clinical results but also changes the patient experience by encouraging increased independence, self-determination, and participation in self-care. Artificial intelligence (AI)-powered algorithms forecast the course of diseases, wearable technology provides real-time symptom monitoring, and virtual reality creates new opportunities for therapy and rehabilitation. These developments not only lead to better patient outcomes but also lessen the strain on caregivers by offering resources and assistance to those who are essential to the care process.

A Request for Further Innovation, Study, and Advocacy

It's obvious that our adventure with Parkinson's therapy is far from ended as we look to the future. Sustained innovation, research, and lobbying are necessary to propel advancement and surmount impending obstacles. Building on the successes of the past, we need to intensify our efforts in order to better understand Parkinson's disease, provide more potent therapies, and eventually find a cure.

Cooperation and funding from many fields are needed to advance Parkinson's research, from basic science to clinical trials and beyond. In order to bring about significant change, it necessitates the involvement of patients and caregivers in clinical trials, research projects, and advocacy campaigns. In addition, it calls for the dedication of legislators, medical professionals, and business executives to support Parkinson's disease research first, encourage creativity, and guarantee fair access to care for all PD patients.

In conclusion, the battle against Parkinson's disease is entering a new phase marked by hope and healing. Millions of people impacted by this difficult condition could have their lives completely changed if we work together with unyielding dedication. Let us work together to advance scientific knowledge, support people who are affected by Parkinson's disease, and envision a time when the disease will not only be treated but completely eradicated—a time filled with promise for a world free of Parkinson's disease.